The Six P's of Physician Leadership

A Primer for Emerging and Developing Leaders

D1293271

Bruce Flareau, MD

J.M. Bohn

Foreword by

Daniel J. VanDurme, MD

This publication is intended to provide accurate and authoritative information in regard to the subject. Statements and opinions expressed are those of the authors.

ISBN: 0-98-999810-X
ISBN-13: 978-0-9899981-0-9

Kumu Press
5847 Long Bayou Way South
St. Petersburg, Fl 33708
707-992-5868
kumupress@gmail.com
www.kumupress.com

Special Orders. Discounts are available on quantity purchases of 10 or more copies. Please contact Kumu Press Sale at the above address.

The Six Ps of Physician Leadership. A Primer for Emerging and Developing Leaders / Bruce Flareau and J.M. Bohn p. cm.

ABOUT THE AUTHORS

Bruce Flareau, MD, is President of BayCare Physician Partners, a clinically integrated network in the Tampa Bay area with 1,200 physicians. He also leads clinical leadership and quality teams as the Executive Vice President of Physician Affairs at BayCare Health System, in the Tampa Bay area of Florida.

Dr. Flareau has been a national and international speaker on a variety of health care topics, including clinical, academic, administrative, information technology, leadership development and healthcare reform. He has also authored a variety of published books, articles and book chapters. Most recently, he co-authored the book, "Clinical Integration, A Roadmap to Accountable Care," which is now in its second edition.

Before becoming a full-time physician executive, Dr. Flareau spent more than 20 years as a practicing family physician. He has been recognized as a full professor at two universities and has served as a residency program director and director of medical education.

He is a certified physician executive, and a fellow of the American Academy of Family Physicians and the American College of Physician Executives.

Dr. Flareau was awarded the Robert Graham Physician Executive Award from the American Academy of Family Physicians in 2012.

He obtained his medical degree from State University of New York, Upstate Medical Center, Syracuse, and completed his Family Medicine Residency at Bayfront Medical Center in Florida. He was born in New York and currently lives in St. Petersburg, Fla., with his wife and two daughters.

J.M. Bohn. We are all on a journey. Early career experience in junior management for a large defense contractor in the late 90s provided lessons in leadership that were applied later when elected as president of the Tampa Junior Chamber of Commerce in 2003. Over the following two years Jo collaboratively led a 10-member board of directors with fellow young professionals from the private sector, government agencies, and not-for-profit organizations who worked together to triple the size of the volunteer organization and its contributions to the Tampa Bay community. Jo grew to understand the importance of servant leadership as discussed by Joseph Jaworski, in *Synchronicity. The Inner Path of Leadership.* 14 years in the defense industry and U.S. Navy followed by the last seven years in the healthcare industry focused on quality, technology innovation, and care transformation.

With an MBA completed in 2006, in 2013 Jo is a doctoral student in the University of Louisville School of Public Health and Information Sciences and principal for KMI Communications, LLC (www.km4i.com) with published works that include:

- Co-author of *M.D. 2.0. Physician Leadership for the Information Age* (2012),

- Co-author of *Accountable Care. A Roadmap for Success, First Ed.* (2011),

- Co-author of *Clinical Integration. A Roadmap to Accountable Care, Second Ed.* (2011),

- Author of *Your Next Steps... in Healthcare Transformation* (2011).

Self-improvement is a continual focus of Jo's life with a passion for how to lead others through transformational change in careers and life.

CONTENTS

ACKNOWLEDGMENTS

Bruce Flareau, M.D.

The rudiments of this book began when my faculty and I were training resident family physicians in the early 1990s and realized the need for a leadership development curriculum. We had young minds to shape and provide the necessary leadership fundamentals for, yet we found very little on the topic intended specifically for physicians. Oliver Oyama, PA, PhD Psychology, and Jeff Sourbeer, MD, worked with me as we slowly hatched the multi-"P" concept of leadership. Initially, only four then five and later six P's came into being.

Others have offered additional P's but often they seemed redundant with what had already been characterized. I am indebted to Oliver and Jeff as astute colleagues and educators who helped gel this idea of physician leadership. I am also indebted to Jo Bohn a friend, colleague and co-author of other works, who encouraged me to carry on and finish this book. Similarly Terry Bradley, MD, and Hal Ziecheck, MBA are trusted colleagues who helped me in my own career development and encouraged the development of this literary work. My wife Kathy and daughters Danielle and Christine have given me the strength to write and the fortitude to learn from my life experiences as well as from others.

Without their support and encouragement this body of work would still be a slide deck or perhaps just a concept.

J.M. Bohn

This opportunity to collaborate with Dr. Flareau on this book and other past works is appreciated. My career experience at BayCare Health System served as a paradigm shifting place in my life and career. It was an extension of my graduate school experience and an immersion into the challenges experienced in our nation's healthcare system.

To the physicians, nurses, and other healthcare leaders I've had the chance to work with, I extend my thanks. If not for your support and encouragement, my own pursuit about how to manage change and help others would not be possible today.

I owe special thanks to Grace Terrell, MD,

who I had the privilege of collaborating with on, *M.D. 2.0.: Physician Leadership in the Information Age. From Hero to Duyukdv.* The work with Dr. Terrell greatly expanded my knowledge of the physician's culture, challenges, and education journey in the twenty-first century and prepared me to co-author this work with Dr. Flareau.

FOREWORD

The Six P's of Physician Leadership

Daniel J. Van Durme, MD, FAAFP

Physicians cannot underestimate the importance of acquiring and perfecting leadership skills. Virtually every physician is a leader, whether in a private practice, an operating room, or an emergency room. Within a community, physicians are seen as leaders in a wide range of issues involving health and other human services. Some may choose to be leaders, while others may be pushed or pulled into leadership positions within healthcare systems or within the life of a community. The principles laid out in this book will provide a framework for building the essential skills needed by novice leaders, as well as a framework for the reflection and growth of experienced leaders.

Do we need yet another book on leadership? Do physicians who are already chronically behind on reading medical journals and reports, not to mention reading for pleasure or personal growth, really need another book to read? The answer is absolutely YES! Flareau and Bohn have put together a brief, yet substantial, primer on the essential aspects of leadership that directly apply to all physicians and physicians-in-training.

Volumes of books have been written on just one of the "P's"—such as "People" or "Process"—but I have yet to encounter any that capture virtually all of the key aspects of leadership in manageable pieces. Reading one chapter every few days gives the reader a chance to reflect and apply the information in their unique workplace. It can serve to stimulate dialogue with co-workers or other colleagues in areas in which we may have our own strengths and weaknesses.

The authors use pragmatic and timely advice for the twenty-first century physician working in an ever-changing environment. With digestible, yet thought-provoking pieces on issues ranging from attention to one's "virtual presence" in email and social media, to maintaining a proper work-life balance, the reader will find practical value throughout the text.

This book serves as a "primer" in multiple ways. It is an elementary or introductory book that gives early learners an overview of the core concepts of a subject. In another sense, this book can "prime the pump" that starts the flow of ideas and behaviors that can make any physician a more effective leader.

Read, reflect, and implement the lessons in this book. Engage others to do the same. The healthcare system needs excellent physician leaders more than ever before.

Daniel J. Van Durme, MD, FAAFP

Professor and Chair, Department of Family Medicine and Rural Health Director, Center on Global Health Florida State University College of Medicine

INTRODUCTION

Don't just do something, stand there.

Through the years, we have observed a number of leaders emerge and succeed where others have either failed or never reached their potential. Yet other would-be leaders have stopped short of rising to the occasion of engagement at all. So what is it amongst these individuals that set them apart from one another? What are the competencies of leadership and can they be learned?

Leadership is often talked about and countless quotes and anecdotes exist. However, in the physician realm, there are minimal resources directed to their unique circumstances. A global health care system that is rapidly evolving in the digital age will require more physician leaders to champion organizational transformation across the global healthcare landscape.

It has been said that physicians are in the top 1% of educated human beings and thus clearly physicians are smart. However, as we discuss in the chapters to follow, being smart alone does not make for a good leader. In addition, physicians have been regarded for their clinical acumen and one-to-one relationship capabilities or even their academic prowess. Again, these attributes do not solely make for a good leader.

Training Future Physician Leaders

Medical schools have historically selected physicians for their intelligence but paid far less attention to relationship management, emotional intelligence and other considerations that would constitute great leadership. While we are starting to make the turn to put more focus on these critical needs for future physician leaders in academia, there is a need for an industry level renaissance to support systemic challenges and the need to cultivate leadership essentials in current and future physician leaders. Previously little time has been spent cultivating what did exist in these other areas. In fact, a 2011 Health Affairs article entitled, *Gaps in Residency Training Should be Addressed to Better Prepare Doctors For a Twenty-First-Century Delivery System*, discussed gaps in training or deficiencies of new graduate physicians (per a survey of Kaiser Permanente clinical department chiefs in 2010). A few of which were cited as:[i]

- Continuity of care,

\- Background with health information technologies (health IT),

\- Leadership and management skills,

\- Systems thinking.

This is coupled with the March 2013 Physician Executive article, *A Call for Physician Leadership at All Levels*, that identified the national urgency for the need for more physician leaders to be readied for leading systems and teams.[ii]

So we find ourselves with a large workforce of physicians in whom little leadership development energies have collectively been applied, yet we are at a time in our history where physician leadership is critical to our future.

Health care reform predicts and even requires that we move from a cottage industry of providers to one of "big medicine", from a workforce of doers to leaders. Outsourcing this to consultants and third party facilitators may satisfy some of the needs, but until it is baked into the cultural DNA of the industry, it will require great care and feeding for sustainability.

Individual physicians will need to see the

need to learn and develop these skills.

The Six P's and Structure of This Book

The *Six P's of Physician Leadership* is a body of work that begins to answer these questions in an easy to understand way. It lays out concepts that existing leaders, up and coming leaders, and potential leaders can incorporate in their daily initiatives.

The *Six P's of Physician Leadership* are:

People	Process
Presence	Perspective
Politics	Principles of Business

In this book we will explore each of the P's in unequal amounts and raise your awareness of their relevance to physician leadership. Unequal amounts because some components are well covered elsewhere and need only be referenced, while others need great expanding, in particular from the physician perspective. Much of this book is written from experience gained as a physician and that of a strategist who has worked to understand the essence of the dilemmas and challenges faced by physicians in the transition from the cottage industry of the twentieth-century to today's evolving clinically integrated care delivery environment.

Becoming a leader and remaining a great leader is a personal journey of self-development with its own inherent obstacles, opportunities and discipline. It all begins with self-awareness and much of this writing is intended to focus in that realm.

So let us begin with one of the most important P's—People.

Bruce Flareau, MD, FAAFP, FACPE, CPE

J.M. Bohn, MBA

October 2013

PEOPLE

Relationship management, the key to success.

Building the Team

The process of creating an effective and cohesive multidisciplinary team starts with a leader having the resolve to determine who the key players and team members should be. Decisions and selection of team members are made one person at a time and as such your ability to influence decisions is dependent upon your ability to form meaningful relationships with others. The nature of those relationships begins with how you view the world and how well you can interact with the people in it. Cultivating relationships with people, working through conflicts, preventing issue escalation, and negotiating mutual benefits are key ingredients of successful relationship management and effective leadership. In the life cycle of business relations, being able to influence decisions comes through the creation of coalitions and advocates who see the need for change.

Steven Covey, in the *Seven Habits of Highly Effective People* points out that interdependence with others is the highest form of victory. In this classic teaching he stresses ways to cultivate relationships and influence management that strive for win-win outcomes, by seeking first to understand before being understood, and finally looking for synergies with key stakeholders.

Each of these issues represents elements of relationship management that can strengthen or hinder our abilities as a leader in working with people. In this chapter some key points will be made about starting, maintaining, and ending relationships in a positive and productive manner. Having an understanding of the importance of relationships leads to the ultimate goal of building high-performing teams.

Jim Collins, in his book *Good to Great,* teaches us that in order to be effective leaders you must "get the right people on the bus."[iii] This act of selecting the right people emphasizes the need to have skills and knowledge in working with others. In Collins' book he points out that with the right people, you can address nearly any problem or issue and can turn your bus as the need arises.

In selecting or cultivating "the right people" it is imperative that we look beyond the hard skills of intelligence quotient (IQ) and job competence as a tactician. Instead we look at the emotional intelligence quotient (EQ) as the key ingredient. EQ refers to your ability to see, analyze, interact, and control emotions. It goes beyond the 'what' of getting the 'right answer' and instead speaks to the 'how' or the way in which you arrive at that answer. This is the people factor of great leaders and your own EQ is the primary determinant of your ability to lead.

Steven Covey's son wrote in *The Speed of Trust*, that we learn that trust is a key ingredient in human interaction with enormous implications on our effectiveness as leaders.[iv] In this writing, Covey points out that to earn trust you must first extend smart trust to others. It is how you treat those around you. Goethe once said, "treat people as if they were what they ought to be and you help them become what they are capable of being." Behaviors such as this earn trust. Remember that as physician leaders and as clinicians you are only as good as your reputation. What took years to earn can be lost in minutes or even seconds.

As we consider the human interaction and our interdependence on people, various considerations come to light. For example, to be a great leader, do you have to be friends with the people you lead? Is friendship a necessary element of developing mutual trust and respect? Most would argue that friendship is not a necessary ingredient. Yet, as with most things, the polar opposite is not a healthy place to be either. Creating enemies does not engender a sense of trust but rather creates winners and losers. Instead, great leaders look to build credibility through open and honest communication. For example, take the scenario of a mother who wants to be a great parent. Does she need to dress as though 20 years younger and befriend the child to be a credible and effective parent? Again, many would see that as over compensation. Children want their parents to be their parents just as followers want their leaders to be leaders. This is not to say you should not form friendships or even avoid friendships, but rather is intended to help you start to define the role and help your own decision making as you develop your critical thinking skills as a leader.

Relationships

So let us turn to three specific components of relationships: forming new relationships, ending old relationships and maintaining existing relationships.

New Relationships

First is forming new relationships. As a leader who do you need to interact with to become more effective? Are there movers and shakers in your community, your specialty society, your legislative region, your local hospitals or elsewhere that it would behoove you to form a relationship with? If so, do you know who they are? Have you ever reached out to them to introduce yourself?

Senior leaders have no reservation about forming relationships and exploring possibilities with others. For example, the entire legislative process is often dependent upon one-on-one relationships that congressmen and senators have trusted experts in whom they can rely upon when an issue arises.

Covey would call this "depositing in the emotional bank account." Here we simply see it as good relationship management. Of course, don't be arrogant and certainly don't waste people's time, but do reach out to others to at least make their acquaintance. One cautionary note regarding this issue of forming new relationships. We are not asking you to be something you are not, nor to reach out to people you have no desire of working with. Be true to yourself and your instincts. People can see through phony or contrived initiatives, and it is better to forego a relationship than to force one where you would rather not have one.

Ending Relationships

Ending relationships is as important as forming new ones. You will be remembered by how you function when things are other than ideal. If you become bitter, disparaging, and ugly with someone, those around you will lose confidence. Alternatively if you handle the transition with dignity and respect, those behaviors will not go unnoticed by others. People will come to trust you more and this virtue is critical to your success as a leader. Remember, the world is smaller than you might imagine. "Till whence we meet again," is a phrase that may surprise you. Why needlessly burn bridges when parting ways with someone. Even terminating an employee can have a professionally reasonable outcome much of the time. Giving formative feedback as to why there may be a mismatch between the job needs and an employee or team member's level of performance can sometimes be viewed as a relief.

You don't have to denigrate someone just because they are not fulfilling a certain job or completing an assigned task. If placed in a different role or under different circumstances they may perform admirably. Separate their performance from your feedback about them as a person or individual. This presumes that you previously conveyed the performance expectations in an understandable manner, set clear targets and gave the individual the opportunity to exceed your expectations. If done well, you will mutually come to the same conclusion and preserve both parties integrity much, although not all of the time. Even in those times where it goes poorly, those around you will see the extremes of your efforts to make it right and again you will be supported by your team.

A classic work on business relationships is *Crucial Conversations,* by Kerry Patterson and colleagues.[v] Sitting down with people and having a difficult discussion on performance expectations, behavior or organizational disagreements is not easy, fun, nor wanted. But it is absolutely essential for a great leader to be able to handle these situations when they arise - and they will.

Maintaining Relationships

As introduced earlier, maintaining relationships is not an accidental venture. Often people will spot you some latitude when you first meet. However, there are some details that a trusted partner would be expected to learn over time with someone who matters. For example, do you know what the other individual prefers to be called?

Too often a mispronounced name or the presumption that an abbreviated nickname is acceptable sets a relationship into a downward spiral. Assuming that Charles is ok with Chuck, or that Kimberly is OK with Kim is presumptuous and disrespectful at best. Instead ask people what they want to be called and use their preferred name. If you forget, acknowledge it and ask again. Keep notes in your contact list if you need to as no one can remember everything. Many physicians have done this for years with their patients, but seem to miss the mark when working administratively.

This small gesture, asking how someone prefers to be referred to, can open doors and demonstrate you to be a caring and compassionate individual who invests in people. Being labeled a people person is a good thing when it comes to leadership. Similarly, do you know how people like to be recognized? Do they cherish public acclaim, prestige, private recognition, time, or money? Knowing what they value and using that as part of their reward system, is far more effective than the latter. Getting a pair of baseball tickets if you don't like baseball is not a motivator.

So as you develop a team, whether it is your office staff, administrative staff, or something larger, remember to explore issues such as their preferred name, preferred motivation, and their likes and dislikes. As we learned from Collins, getting the right people on your bus is critical to you success and striving to create positive healthy relationships will strengthen efforts to make organizational progress.

Creating sweatshops does not lend itself to highly functioning teams. Instead, to have a high performing team you must invest in the people around you and give them opportunities to exceed expectations. Like parenting, it is hard to be around solely for those times that are later deemed quality time. Instead, if you are around enough, some of that time will be viewed as quality.

What have you done to create quality time with your team? Do you listen actively, have an open door policy, or expend energies to create interactive times with those around you? Listening actively to your clinical and administrative team members will mean a few things:

- Giving them your undivided attention,

- Withholding your own comments until they have had a chance to fully express their opinions, and

- Taking the time to evaluate and process a considerate response.

As you consider these issues, ponder too your own attributes, likes and dislikes. What makes you the right person to drive the bus? Why are you viewed differently than your peers? Do you listen well? Are you thoughtful in your demeanor? Are you a content expert?

Answering these questions can help each of us understand ourselves better and can involve serious introspective and reflective thought about what makes us tick. Bill George in his 2007 book, *True North. Discovering Your Authentic Leadership*, wrote,

> "Knowing yourself can be compared to peeling back the layers of an onion as you search for your true self."[vi]

As much as we work toward putting standards in place in the processes we implement in healthcare, each of us as leaders are unique. With this uniqueness, comes a differing degree of self-awareness that helps us know and understand our strengths, weaknesses, and interpersonal challenges. Some people choose to ignore the perspective and perception (a topic to be expanded upon in the next chapter) that others have of them and are OK with that, but the introspective and compassionate leader will recognize the importance of perception and balance it with *self-admonition* to be better leaders and more helpful to those we help and serve on a daily basis.

When tending to personal relationships, a question often pondered relates to personal disclosures. Does story telling of personal activities make the leader a better leader or should the leader keep a professional separation between work and home life? To some extent personal disclosures are a personal matter and there is no one correct answer. However, to never talk about yourself or your personal pursuits could be to create a disconnected and somewhat aloof environment. Conversely, only talking about yourself and your family can be viewed as bragging, taking advantage of others or just plain rude.

Self Disclosure

So where does a great leader land on the matter of personal disclosure? Humility is a virtue and personal disclosures with an emphasis on humility are often the preferred approach. Telling stories about your trip to Fiji, unless solicited, can create barriers to meaningful and effective team development and effective leaders have effective teams.

Story telling is a powerful tool and is not to be dismissed. Use it to establish culture and engender meaning and direction for your organization or purpose. Use it to humanize yourself and make yourself approachable by people who matter to you. Often great leaders seem bigger than life and approachability is something to be cultivated and maintained. Self-disclosure reminds people that you are human, you make mistakes and that you value their input as a friend and colleague.

Leading Teams Through Change

One of the most challenging issues for leaders at any stage of their career today is leading their teams and organizations through periods of change. Transformation is being caused by several factors but three *societal ecosystem factors* to touch on are shown in Figure 1-1.

Figure 1-1. Societal Ecosystem Factors Effecting Change

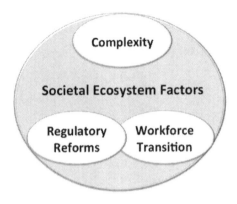

People in every healthcare organization are touched by these three factors.

Complexity—The U.S. healthcare system has evolved as a complex adaptive system. The intricacies of the system involve independent agents, feedback loops, non-linear relationships and the occurrence of unintended adverse consequences that result from systemic change. People are impacted positively or negatively by complexity factors that can lead to unforeseen changes. In light of this factor, leaders need to be prepared to handle rapidly emerging issues that affect their teams.

Regulatory Reforms—The impact of cyclical regulatory reforms have brought about significant changes that affect each generation of patients, physicians and the healthcare organizations as they evolve. Reform efforts have been occurring throughout the last two centuries and are certain to be part of the physician leader's landscape of issues to contend with for decades to come. Managing the changes initiated by regulatory reforms and understanding how they affect a leader's team and organization is essential.

Workforce Transition—The aging of the Baby Boomer segment of our population is not only a patient issue but also a workforce issue for physician leaders to be constantly aware of in today's environment. As the workforce ages there will be new challenges to address in terms of staffing shortages, technology impacts, workflow, and communication changes for physician leaders to address with their next generation teams as their organizations move forward.

There are several theories and processes for managing change but a few key tenets for physician leaders to remember are:

- Recognize the signs and need to prepare your team for change early in any process or scenario.

- Have a clear vision and roadmap for how to lead your team to their new destination albeit geographic or functional.

- Plan to measure and evaluate progress along the way and after any significant change is instituted.

Physician leaders are facing greater scrutiny and accountability for their efforts today than at any time in history. As your own leadership journey unfolds understand the importance of adaptability to the changing environment.

Leaders Develop People. People Make the Leader.

As we close this discussion around people remember the words of Ralph Waldo Emerson when he said,

"…to leave the world a bit better, whether by a healthy child, a garden patch or a redeemed social condition; to know that even one life has breathed easier because you lived—that is to have succeeded."

Successful leaders know this well and take it to heart each and every day.

PRESENCE

"Character is much easier kept than recovered."

Thomas Paine

1737-1809

English-American Political Activist and Theorist

Impressions

Unlike the first P, which speaks to how you view and interact with others, the second P relates to how they view you. It is your reputation in their minds eye. Do you know how others view you? Will anyone tell you? Are you empathic or erratic, sincere, or psychotic, rational or ruthless, caring, or uncaring, trustworthy or otherwise?

Your presence is determined by non-verbal and verbal communication—through actions, mannerisms, off the record commentary, appearances, voice and incidental encounters. Are you moody? Do you think before you speak? Do you listen and try first to understand? Are you confident in your demeanor?

In my own development as a physician leader I learned early on that I have a strong personality that can hamper my approachability. My presence was strong and at times made me unapproachable. It took some honest feedback to realize that often when I am deep in thought, I furrow my brow and can appear angry. An interesting observation since I am rarely if ever an angry person—yet perception is reality. While I worked on not furrowing my brow, as I did not want to stop deep thinking and problem solving, the other thing I did was self-disclose this perceptual quirk. I learned to poke fun at it, orient others to it, and in doing so, made myself more approachable and a better leader. It all started with insight and honest communication.

As a leader, understanding and developing your presence is essential. Too often physicians come forward, passionate around an issue, and become viewed as zealots, irrational, or extremist. This lowers your influence opportunities and is frustrating to say the least.

An Executive Persona

Great leaders either naturally or through learned behavior have what has been deemed an *executive persona or being presidential.*

The art of maintaining an executive persona is a way to manage your reputation, convey understandable messages and further your effectiveness as a leader. Being presidential is just as it implies—what would a president do or say in this circumstance? How do you walk the moral and ethical high ground? What words or actions would connote a different presence?

Cultivating this type of behavior is to realize that as a leader you are never "off the record." Everything you do and say is a reflection of your character. If the president of the United States was found intoxicated on the White House steps yelling racial slurs or demeaning commentary, his or her political career would be severely hampered. Confidence would be lost in such a leader and the same is true of other leaders in other positions of authority. Instead society wants an honest law abiding leader who perpetually walks the moral high ground, is not above the law, who speaks with passion and conviction, viewed as fair, articulate, firm when needed, and the purveyor of all that is good and righteous.

Of course, no leaders can be all things to all people, but certain proven leadership behaviors can be demonstrated and are worth your effort. Maintaining an executive persona can be hard to understand but people know it when they see it.

Diplomacy

In today's U.S. and global health care environment, teamwork among physicians, consultants, and senior management is playing a key role in ensuring that key decisions include comprehensive clinical, financial, and administrative perspectives. As the health care system continues to undergo change, physicians are entering the path of consultancy work. We have had the good fortune of witnessing this essential trait at work and embodied by some executive level physician consultants who clearly demonstrated having a *diplomatic presence*.

Knowing what to say, how to say it, and when to say it, is something that typically takes years of experience to grasp. For those junior physicians seeking this career path, understand the importance of patience, fact-finding, and drawing upon clinical evidence along with developing your own personal tactfulness for presenting information relevant for key decision-making by leaders and clients.

Let us consider two additional scenarios to gain a deeper understanding of this notion of presence. In particular, presence *in person* and presence in *cyberspace*. Each realm has its own intricacies including a list of do's and don'ts relative to evolving your presence.

Presence in Person

So, how are you viewed in meetings by your staff and by the people who clean your office? Do you know?

As a leader, you are only as good as your reputation! Yes, write that down and commit it to memory. Your reputation is paramount to your success as a leader and a great reputation is hard earned and easily lost. As such a great leader must realize that he or she is never off stage. As mentioned above, a stellar reputation as a great leader and statesman of a highly moral and ethical character would all but be destroyed in a matter of seconds with cavalier "off the record" commentary. Your inner character does not change before or after work. J.C. Watts is quoted as saying, "Character is doing the right thing when nobody is looking."

There are too many people who think that the only thing that's right is to get by, and the only thing that's wrong is to get caught. And so it is with your *in person* presence. You don't know what tidbit of information someone will use to judge your character. Perhaps you were recovering from a recent illness and made certain facial grimaces unrelated to a conversation but left the other party with a misimpression. Think of how U.S. presidents are put under the microscope and analyzed for their attire, hand gestures, tone of their voice, oh, and of course the choice of their words. All of these things culminate in the notions for which others formulate opinions around your leadership qualities.

Many instruments have been developed to assess how others see us and what our default personality traits are. Myers Briggs personality inventory and DISC profiles (Dominance, Influence, Steadiness, and Conscientiousness) are tools to help objectify these traits and behaviors. Whatever method or tool you choose, recognize that there are two ways in which to be effective as a leader. You can be feared or you can be respected. The former is a style that has worked for many leaders who have had successful careers and been held by highly feared individuals. Yet questions remain as to how far this style can truly take a leader and whether or not it is intrinsically fulfilling.

More aligned with ethical and effective leadership is the notion of leading with and from a position of respect. As a staff sergeant in World War II, my father Donald G. Flareau, told me how he "never asked someone to do something he himself would not do." His men respected him for his convictions and many gave their lives on the battlefield—character like that is inspiring to say the least. Notice, however that earning respect can be an isolated activity or a re-occurring one. A martyr may be respected for figuratively jumping on a grenade; however, this is a onetime event from which recovery is often not possible. A leader who openly engages in a needless confrontational debate, may feel good in the moment but lose the trust of other leaders in the process.

So where do people draw their information to formulate opinions about your character? Perhaps it's from articles, overhearing conversations and other indirect resources. Or from consult notes, office staff commentary, or even desk clerks. Ask yourself, do you have an opinion upon the moral convictions or character of Bill Gates? Princess Diana? Michael Jackson? If so, from what sources of information did you draw your conclusions?

The answer is typically, yes you have an opinion and it is firmly based upon indirect and flawed sources of information. Yet you still have an opinion and you are no different than anyone else. Your *in person* presence is your perpetual opportunity to reaffirm who you are and the true nature of your character.

Presence in Cyber Space

What happens in Vegas stays in social media forever.

With the advent of the Internet, mass communication, social media, and one-to-many asynchronous communication is all about us, and so too is a virtual presence of who you are perceived to be in cyber space. As a leader, should this matter? Should you separate out the professional you from the personal you? Of course, to some extent, this is a matter of personal preference, and no matter what you decide, there are ways to mitigate and shape your virtual presence.

Email

First, how should you handle email communication? Here style matters a great deal. Length of message, font selection, punctuation and even color all convey meaning, whether favorable or unfavorable. Sanserif (e.g., Times New Roman for example) font is best for print or print-equivalent media in terms of ease of reading. Block font (e.g., Arial for example) is best used for projected media. Hence Sanserif font is the way to go for most email. All capitals or all bolded fonts convey shouting and should be avoided unless that is your intention.

In terms of writing style, starting an email with who, what, where, when or how can be read as accusatory. The same can be said of starting with you or I. Email length also tells a story about your character. Do you send multi-paragraph emails? If the answer is yes, would it be more appropriate to have called the individual? I have learned through the years that if my email is getting past a paragraph, the better part of valor is to delete the message and get on the phone. Alternatively emails that are too cryptic can be viewed as terse or disrespectful. While these may be efficient, the omission of pleasantries such as hello, thank you, or please, can mistakenly convey the wrong message.

So when it comes to the length of your message, think of email as a convenient way in which to efficiently convey short single point messages. Don't be too long, or too short, but rather just right. Remember to sign your email and use color sparingly so as not to detract from the purpose of the message. If all this sounds too complex, take a look at the following example.

HENRY – WHERE IS THE REPORT YOU PROMISED ME THE OTHER DAY?

Compare that to the following:

Hi Henry - just checking in regarding the report we discussed the other day. Are we still good? Bruce

Can you see the difference in terms of tone? The first looks to be an accusatory shouting while the second is a collegial inquiry. Don't be the victim of meaning one and connoting the other.

On a related note, we need to consider the use of blind and un-blind copying as well as the reply-to-all feature commonly found in email applications. Blind copying is fraught with problems and should routinely be avoided. Think of a scenario where you are sending a note to someone and you don't want them to know you are sending it to someone else. Just the concept reeks of secrecy and mistrust. What if the blinded party forwards that message to the unknowing original recipient? What does that mean in terms of your credibility? For different reasons the "cc" function should often be avoided as well. If the message is important enough to send, shouldn't you purposefully direct it to the intended party? The copy function might be utilized for a secretary in terms of a calendar inquiry, or perhaps an administrative staff, but beyond that it should be used judiciously. Over utilization of this conveys a sense that you don't value those parties enough to purposefully direct the message or to sort through the messages well enough to avoid wasting their time.

Finally the *reply all* function. Clearly there are times when replying to a group makes sense. An interactive online discussion can be held with a team that is comfortable with one another. However, in less comfortable circumstances, replying to all can be viewed as covering your hindquarters and perhaps disrespectful of others at times. Despite the way that information is interpreted, the final point is that people will occasionally interpret electronic communications in ways other than how you intended them. This is the real take home message. Be aware of this downfall, treat others as you would have them treat you, and be mindful of how you use or overuse email. By the way, if you were born after 1990 email is already a dead communication tool. Instant messaging and social media have overtaken it as a vehicle of communication.

So what about Facebook, Hulu, tweeting, and other forms of social media? Can you publish family pictures and jokes on your home page? Recall that whatever you post is essentially in the public domain and will influence opinion around your character. If you don't want to see it on the evening news, the general rule of thumb would be don't post it to the Internet. Many companies maintain social media sites that are business specific. This is a reasonable activity although the sites should be monitored in some fashion. Many human resources departments, hiring authorities, intelligence agencies, news agencies and even attorneys search social media sights when investigating individuals. Keep this in mind the next time you think about posting something.

Understand and Tend to Your Presence

In summary, your presence is your perceived character and therefore essential to your reputation. It is the single most important consideration for leaders to self-monitor and maintain awareness of about themselves.

Many top leaders have hired acting coaches, voice coaches and executive coaches to assist them with their presence. Dressing for success, interview techniques and public speaking seminars are but a limited sample of the kinds of activities that have been developed to assist leaders with this ingredient of success. Given its importance, the wise leader will rank this essential leadership element as a high priority to maintain their *in person* and *virtual* presence.

POLITICS

"For every action there is an equal and opposite reaction."

Sir Isaac Newton

1642-1727

English physicist

Influence

For many physicians, politics has a negative connotation, often viewed with reservation or frank disdain. Yet politics is more about influencing people and is simply a thread in the fabric of every effective leader. The new leader may for example, only rely upon formal reporting structures in order to accomplish work. More experienced leaders will recognize that informal politically influential opinion leaders must also be considered. As with most things, excess reliance upon political acumen is to be avoided, yet complete avoidance is likewise unhealthy. The first order of business is to acknowledge there are political influences in nearly every aspect of what you will do as a leader. Second, is to identify where those influences lie and manage them to the best of your ability. To do anything other than this would be to risk becoming a casualty of political neglect.

As you meet and interact with individuals, and work to influence and shape agendas in some fashion, remember that others will be doing likewise. Ignoring this factor, or solely "walking the high road" assuming the other issues will take care of themselves, is to be naïve and to place yourself at risk. Instead, the politically astute leader tends to the informal communication network, forms personal relationships that keep him or her attuned to alternate opinions, and manages emergent issues proactively. For nearly every opinion or decision point there is usually one or more people with differing opinions. If those belong to opinion leaders, your ability to effect change is that much more difficult. Early identification and proactive intervention are good uses of time and effort in tending to these types of occurrences.

Let us look at an example to drive this point home. Imagine that you are the newly elected chief of staff of a mid-sized hospital, and that one of your new responsibilities is to discipline a high referral physician colleague. You have a professional working relationship with the individual and are aware that he is sometimes abrupt and condescending to staff, and difficult to work with. However, you greatly respect his clinical opinion and he sends you a large number of patients for which you are grateful. Previously you tended to look the other way regarding his behavior, but now in your position of leadership you must enter a letter in his file and subject him to some disciplinary process based upon a recent event. In addition, he is very "connected" with the local medical society as they see him as a renegade who protects their well being when dealing with 'big business.' He has a history of blowing things out of proportion and history tells you that any disciplinary action taken with him may be exaggerated and used to create tensions between the local society and the medical staff.

Just recognizing these factors alone, places you in good stead. Less experienced leaders might either miss these points or knowingly just let the chips fall where they may. While there is no one way to address these complex issues, having the insight that they exist, and forming meaningful relationships of mutual trust and respect, will help you as you move along in such matters. While not an easy task, an experienced leader will have developed a reputation of being fair and just, and will treat this physician with the respect they deserve. Sitting him down, listening to his side of the story, while remaining on point with your message around what constitutes acceptable behavior, are essential elements of what needs to happen in this scenario. Making sure key leaders, either formal or informal are aware of the factual basis for the coaching, while not breaching the physicians own confidence, are political factors of influence that will flank any misdirection that this physician might attempt to create.

Empowerment

While great leaders understand the political nature of people, they also understand the need to let people find their own way. Trying to manage everything for everyone is an exercise in futility. Knowing which issues need intervention and which do not is the job of leadership. Thomas Jefferson is quoted as saying,

> "In matters of style, swim with the current; in matters of principle, stand like a rock."

This is good council in terms of interacting with people on a variety of levels. Both when delegating work through authority or when interacting with others through influence, it is a good rule of thumb to let people internalize and manage the work in their own way; that is, unless it is directionally incorrect from a visioning and outcomes perspective.

Strategic vs. Tactical

This brings us to a discussion around some distinctions between being tactical versus being strategic. Both have their place yet leadership spends much of its time being strategic. Tactical is a short-term activity and should change to meet local conditions. It is the incremental decisions and actions that get a job done.

Managing the details for other people will soon find you labeled a micromanager and both create frustration and lower job satisfaction of otherwise high performing people. Conversely, strategy is a long-term view of where you are heading. It often involves new interventions as opposed to managing existing activities. Strategy often does not change based upon local conditions as it is larger, more global and all the more impactful for an organization.

Being strategic is the equivalent of *picking your battles*. Aligning your organization and initiatives in ways that matter most is a series of decision points. Like the political process itself, knowing which knob to turn and when, are key attributes that often require experience and mentorship. Sometimes referred to as earning your wings, or *I have the scars to prove it*. Learning to be strategic is not a straight-line activity. Learning that being right and being effective are different steps on the road to a successful leadership experience. That always having the last word, is an unnecessary exploitation of authority and at the end of the day, people want to do good work in ways that matter. Be strategic, be political, and be effective.

Triangulation

In the process of relationship development and honing your political acumen, there is one additional consideration that bears discussion—the concept of *triangulation*. Some might term this conflict avoidance or overzealous use of the political process of influence management. In short, it is the act of working through a third party rather than directly with the individual with whom you have an issue.

Take for example the peer leader who disagrees with a key initiative you wish to implement. Perhaps a committee needs capital funding that requires approval and you know this person does not support you on this issue. Triangulation would have you talking to others to win their favor and influence the decision. To some extent this may be productive, but as uncomfortable as it may be, the better part of valor is to privately sit with the individual, listen until you understand their position, and address the issues directly rather than triangularly.

Admittedly this is not comfortable and conflict management rarely is. However, ask yourself, if the scenario were reversed, how would you want to be treated? Rather than manipulating the committee to get what you want to bring the issue to the forefront, addressing the concerns strategically and walking the high road will serve you better in the long run.

Let us explore a second triangulation scenario that many leaders, wanting to be liked by their colleagues and team members, might easily fall prey to. . Imagine you have an employee who is showing up late, leaving early and slacking while on the job. Others are increasingly frustrated and want you to do something. The other team members want to know that you have disciplined the problem employee and want to know the details. In fact you have seen the performance issues, and privately met with the person and put them on a progressive disciplinary plan that may lead to termination. As much as the rest of the team wants to know that, think to yourself how you would want to be treated. Is it their business to know the details of that coaching? Disciplinary actions are best done directly and have no place in the hallways. As tempting as it would be to explain that you are addressing the problem and elaborating on all the things you are doing, a respected leader will remain confidential and stay the course in silence.

Scratching the itch of interested colleagues to know someone else's business is a short-term tactic to earn relationship points, yet it is a bad strategy. Similarly, always telling the truth without convenient spin or interpretation will serve you best in the long run when it comes to building and maintaining relationships.

Ultimately people realize that if the conditions were different, you would equally breach their own confidence and tell those details to others. While maintaining confidentiality may be hard, it is essential. You will be respected for it and over time, as you resolve the issues, the trust will be stronger.

Embracing Collaboration

In summary, politics is simply the art of influence management. It involves forming alliances, listening intently, understanding the agendas of various stakeholders, and selectively intervening where you see necessary. Being collaboration driven, showing strong business acumen and maintaining both professional will and personal humility are essentials for every leader[vii] and an intentional focus on these facets of your professional development will enhance your abilities to manage and navigate political relations. Engaging in politics is not to be avoided, but rather managed and embraced.

Very little progress of substance happens when we work in a vacuum. Great leaders need people to lead and are intentional in their efforts to engage in the network of their ecosystem to drive relations for the benefit of those they lead.

PROCESS

It is not just the destination but the journey itself that matters.

Awareness in the Moment

Leaders need to understand the means by which their goals and objectives will be achieved. For every activity, program or initiative there are one or more processes with multiple steps that may be required. Processes can be looked at in two ways. The first refers to the ability to examine what is happening around you, sometimes referred to as situational awareness. Second is the discipline of examining current state processes and making them better for the future. Enabling a process improvement that sets the stage for greater efficiency and effectiveness in the future state.

The ability to process a meeting while simultaneously participating in the meeting may seem an odd distinction and yet it is an important one. As a participant in a meeting you are listening and reflecting, you are interpreting information you hear and continually testing that against your own frames of reference. You are in the moment and may be very focused on the content of the discussion or topic at hand.

This is an important attribute and as an isolated skill can be honed for a variety of tasks. For example the lifeguard who needs to ignore extraneous activities and spot the drowning victim, or the airport security officer who needs to look at countless bags and spot the dangerous component of one bag. Conversely, as a meeting facilitator, you have to rise above your own opinions and monitor the room participants in a broader and less defined way. You need to see when people are losing interest, when they are fidgeting, when nonverbal cues are signaling disagreement or unrest.

Great leaders can parallel track and both participate in the meeting while simultaneously processing the meeting. For complex tasks it is often preferential to have a neutral party facilitator, as they can monitor the room, draw out questions, and are not tied to a particular outcome or result. Even so, you should not leave the meeting dynamics entirely to others. Fortunately, situational awareness or "processing" a room can be an acquired skill. Have you ever had the experience of watching a movie or a television program and have no idea that something occurred around you? Perhaps you were so engrossed in the program that you missed another moviegoer in the back row having to be removed from the theater for one reason or another.

If you think that you don't miss anything in a meeting, you might want to watch some version of the gorilla experiment conducted a number of years ago at Harvard as a psychology study. Authors of the book, *The Invisible Gorilla: How Our Intuitions Deceive Us*, and creators of the experiment, Christopher Chabris and Daniel Simons, videotaped a group of people passing a basketball amongst themselves.[viii] The viewer is asked to specifically count the number of passes. Along the way, a person in a gorilla suit walks into the screen, spends several seconds on screen, and walks off. More than half of those who watch the video do not see the gorilla. Fortunately, that means nearly half the people do. Parallel tracking to both be counting the passes and see the gorilla are worthwhile skills and it begins with awareness.

Similarly in the hospital or business setting, debriefing with another party after a meeting is often helpful to begin to identify what you did not see the first time.

Tools and Techniques

The second aspect of process is that of process improvement. Whether it is Continuous Quality Improvement (CQI), Total Quality Management (TQM) or more contemporary terms like Six Sigma or Lean, this perspective of process is about the science of examining processes and making intelligent changes for the better.

A great leader needs to have an understanding of process improvement. Some would argue that you should have Six Sigma black belt type skills. While a general understanding of performance improvement is essential, great leaders do not have to be experts in Six Sigma level process improvement. Others can do the tactical portions of process improvement. However, understanding the basics are foundational requirements in today's dynamically changing environment for being a great leader. What is a root cause analysis, how do you do brainstorming? What is a process control chart? These process improvement tools and techniques and similar fundamentals should be mastered and fortunately countless writings, courses and materials are available on this subject.

Enabling Progress

In short, being process focused invokes a series of dual existence conundrums. Are you in the meeting or are you a processer of the meeting? Are you focusing on an existing process or developing a new one? Are you enabling a process that holds yourself and your organization accountable, or are you leaning towards process steps that enable excuses rather than delivering results?

In closing we discussed two perspectives on processes, both of which are vital. One as a series of actions and the other of a state of awareness and recognizing at what level you are a participant in it. Yes, as a leader you must become comfortable with seemingly disparate paradox activities—it is as much the rule as it is the exception. When processes are implemented or participated in effectively, it can be an enabler of change that helps your hospital, physician practice or patients achieve their goals (e.g., mitigating chronic conditions, reducing cost, or eliminating medical errors). Every great leader should understand this element of success and recognize when to engage or ensure that proper resources are dedicated to solving problems, overcoming barriers, and striving to achieve goals.

PERSPECTIVE

"The optimist sees the donut, the pessimist sees the hole."

Oscar Wilde

1854-1900

English Poet

How You Look At It

Do you have *perspective*? Can you see past your nose? Do you see the greater good? Are you planning for Monday, or ten years from Monday?

Take for example the story of the man who complained that his shoes were ill fit and how he incessantly complained about his misfortune only to one day meet a man with no feet, suddenly his perspective changed.

In the well-acclaimed movie, *Patch Adams*, Robin Williams is asked by a fellow inpatient psychiatric patient, how many fingers he sees while holding his hand in front of his face.

With three extended fingers he quickly says three. Yet the patient says,

> "see what others do not see, look past the fingers, ... choose to see what others do not."

Suddenly Robin Williams sees the fingers out of focus and there appear more fingers. Yes *perspective* is seeing what others choose not to see, but it is also about our own frame of reference.

During a series of health system employee and physician town hall meetings I put up a slide of a large great white shark in crystal clear water only meters behind a loan kayaker. Each time I would ask the audience which one represented the physician and which one represented the health system. Invariably the administrators saw themselves as sitting in the kayak being pursued by the shark as did the physicians; each felt themselves to be the victim. Of course, no such polarity truly exists. Rather it is one's perspective that sets the tone. Great leaders can rise above personal circumstances and look for the greater good. Furthermore, they can help others see that vision and can mobilize teams around those more virtuous activities.

Peter Hackett, MD reached the summit of Mount Everest in 1981. He created the Himalayan Rescue Association in the 1970s, and later the Denali Medical Research Project in Anchorage, Alaska. He is an expert in expedition medicine and extreme situations. In one of his conferences he made the statement that "'Good judgment comes from bad experiences." It is easy to tell a child to do as you say, not as you do, but there is something about learning from life's experiences. Old Salts, or lifetime boaters, each have stories to tell of mishaps on the high seas. The important point is to learn from the experiences and bring that perspective to the room, while having the wherewithal to realize that others will perceive things entirely different based upon their own set of life experiences.

There is no fast track to gaining perspective. Like moving from knowledge to wisdom, it is a learned attribute. Give people room. Give them the benefit of the doubt, and give them the benefit of your experience—have perspective.

Change the Lens and Change the View

In any given situation a leader may view a situation through a variety of lenses. A sociological lens may shed light on key elements of the human behavior in a particular setting. Applying an engineering or systems thinking lens to view the same situation may set the human behavior elements aside and closely examine the elements of the processes, technologies and resources involved to understand the problem and develop proposed solutions.

The lens chosen by each leader should be versatile and remember that to attain a global and comprehensive perspective it may be helpful to examine each situation through more than one lens.

For every great physician leader, there is the need for flexibility and adaptability. Keeping your perspective broad will allow greater vision and understanding of the situation allowing for more impact on the decisions you make in the future.

Trends and Insights

In 2000 Malcolm Gladwell released his best seller, *The Tipping Point. How Little Things Can Make a Big Difference*. In this fascinating work, Gladwell identified three characteristics of paradigm shifting trends that are simple but should be on the radar of both experienced and emerging leaders alike:[ix]

1. Contagiousness,

2. Little causes can have big effects,

3. Change happens not gradually but at one dramatic moment.

We bring this up to make a point of the importance for every leader to maintain a perspective on trends that are occurring in the global space of the healthcare industry and other sectors as they affect the health of the patients you serve. There are a multitude of issues that every leader is faced with but take for example the scenario that has been faced by many in leadership over the past few years on whether or not to establish a public or private accountable care organization (ACO). There are many foundational issues to consider but one is paying attention to the lessons learned from other organizations in the past, understanding the regulatory burdens and the risks (e.g., financial, administrative and clinical) for every leader weighing this decision.

It's important to not get caught up in the contagiousness of what is transpiring throughout the industry but instead to look at the true paradigm shifting elements of the change that is occurring. The need for change has happened not gradually but can be traced back to the paradigm shifting point of moving from a volume-driven to a value-driven care delivery system that is having a profound effect on how we provide, pay for and improve the quality of care delivered.

Age of Reform

In closing this chapter, a final consideration on perspective is that for physician leaders in the twenty-first century there is an ever increasing need to not only maintain, but to champion a patient and customer focus. Health care today is a different ball game as we have seen dramatic change in generational values, the economic realities for patients to obtain high quality care, and many more changes on the way with health care reform.

So for today's physician leaders and those in the next generation being groomed today, it's critical to maintain this patient-centered focus in all that we do. A servant leader approach is one to consider. In Joseph Jaworski's 1996 book entitled, *Synchronicity. The Inner Path of Leadership*, he concluded the final chapter with,

> "…leadership that can bring forth such predictable miracles is more about being than doing. It is about our orientation of character, our state of inner activity."[x]

Changing our orientation of character and checking our egos at the door is what physician leaders have to do for the good of their patients and their communities. Regardless of whether you operate in the United States, Brazil, Dubai, or Scotland—the mission is the same. To save lives and improve the health of those who come to you in need.

Health care reforms are happening on a global scale and the need for physician leaders is great. Maintaining the perspective that change is inevitable and your patient population is of paramount importance in all decisions made as a leader. Technology, laws, people, and organizations will change—the needs of your patients will change with time so keep them as a priority at all times in your own journey into leadership.

PRINCIPLES OF BUISNESS

"To be physician led and professionally managed."

Thomas A. Atchison, Ed.D

President and founder of Atchison Consulting

Rules of the Road

I have been asked by countless physician leaders whether or not to pursue an MBA or some post-graduate degree in business. In years gone by, most physician leaders were promoted from the ranks based upon innate abilities. After all, physicians are a highly intelligent group of people and who better to lead healthcare than this body of professionals? However as the decades have passed, being a good clinician and having a high IQ are, in and of themselves, not enough in the twenty-first century and this digital age of healthcare.

Today's leader needs to have a firm understanding of business and strategy principles.

- What is a cash flow statement?

- What is a business plan?

- What ratios are worth following to understand the health of an organization?

- How are bond ratings done?

- How much cash should we have on hand?

- What communications approach should we take for this event?

- How do we implement and adopt this new technology?

There are many ways to learn business disciplines and strategy areas from self-study, to online university courses to traditional study and executive societies such as the American College of Physician Executives. No matter the forum, the successful leader will inquire, learn and to varying degrees, master these and related topics.

Similarly, common business practice includes not just finance and accounting but a solid understanding of strategic planning.

- Where do you see your organization in three to five years?

- How do you develop a common understanding of that destination?

- What incremental steps should you take to accept the need for change?

Again, these skills may be learned on the job, in the classroom, or more realistically through a combination of both.

Of course, many physicians chose to be physicians because of an inborn desire to help heal the sick and save lives whenever possible. No amount of external influence can force someone to undergo the grueling course of study to reach this pinnacle of education and societal reputation. Instead there must be some inherent desire to pursue this professional destination. This is what makes physicians unique in the health care business arena. A common understanding of the human mind and body, the contemporary understanding of how to relieve pain and suffering, and how to best coach individuals and families to be as healthy as they can, are the cornerstones of physician hood.

To be *physician led* is a powerful statement for any organization. Yet, truly successful organizations will find themselves both physician led and professionally managed.

As a physician leader you do not need to be an expert in finance or compliance, or business development or accounting. Instead you need a general understanding of all those things and a team of professionals who are as good at their jobs as you are at yours.

Importance of Innovations

Healthcare services will continue to evolve as scientific exploration leads to new technologies that continue to improve our diagnostic, treatment, and predictive capabilities. Perhaps one day robotic nanobots will operate on the cellular level and alleviate disease more proactively. Perhaps mass production of medications will become as inexpensive as computer chips, and today's costly interventions will be pennies on the dollar in the future. In Clayton Christensen's 2009 bestseller, *The Innovator's Prescription, A Disruptive Solution for Health Care*, he delineated between disruptive and sustaining innovations. For those new and novel ideas that are ahead of the curve and contribute to paradigm shifts in the field of medical care, we can consider them as disruptive. Clayton identified three elements of disruptive innovations:[xi]

Table 6-1. Elements of Disruptive Innovations

Element	Description
Technological enabler	New technologies that bring new solutions to the forefront.
Business model innovation	Delivery models for putting the new enablers in practice.
Value network	The infrastructure that supports the delivery models and technological enablers.

Every physician leader should maintain their awareness of new innovations in the industry pipeline. For these are the ideas that can lead to improvement in operating efficiency, increased patient satisfaction, and ultimately save patient lives. Leading teams and organizations through the transformation of clinical and administrative practices in the coming decades will require physicians and clinicians to pave the way for better health care—delivered individually but with a focus on the population and nation. Reducing the cost of care and alleviating some of its burden on society as a whole.

Leading with Focus

The principles of business are universal and apply to all industries. But for the physician leader at any stage of their career it's essential to grasp, use and strengthen their knowledge and application of these principles. The field of innovation is critical to follow and monitor for every physician leader as the technology revolution we are all impacted by infiltrates the intricacies of every element of how we practice, pay for, and care for the patients in our community.

The nation is turning to physicians for leadership of the healthcare system in the twenty-first century. Remember the keys of accountability, collaboration, and maintaining awareness of change at all times.

CONCLUSION

"America can lead a transformation of health care, which will create compelling benefits for the health and health care of all citizens." [xii]

Michael E. Porter and Elizabeth Olmsted Teisberg

Redefining Health Care

2006

Moving Forward

Physicians are being called upon to lead in all facets of our nation's healthcare transformation that is happening at an accelerating pace. In his 1984 Pulitzer prize winning work, *The Social Transformation of American Medicine*, Paul Starr noted,

> "...physicians exercise authority over patients, their fellow workers, in health care, and even the public at large in matters within, and sometimes outside, their jurisdiction." [xiii]

Starr's work is over three decades old but

his statement still holds true. Physicians are trained in understanding the biological foundations of human life. With this knowledge comes a level of respect and intrinsic esteem bestowed by society—making the importance of the *Six P's for Physician Leadership* a higher priority as a set of principles to be embraced. The United States is squarely focusing on improving the health of its population. Health reforms, technology innovations, public health programs, and new care delivery models are deployed throughout communities to reduce health disparities, reduce the prevalence of chronic disease, and aid individuals by improving the quality of life for all our citizens.

Leaders set the course for what lies ahead in terms of overcoming challenges and barriers to improve the systems of care that exist today. With this comes needed celebration for the successes, lives saved and quality of lives improved. Along the way it will be the physician leaders who embrace collaboration and forge the pathways and interventions for having healthier communities.

The Journey Begins Now

Throughout this book we have tried to stress the importance of personal balance and your increasing interdependence upon others as a leader. No longer an army of one, the successful physician leader must work with and through others. The *Six P's of Physician Leadership* are intended to raise your awareness and provide a roadmap of discovery as you grow and mature into the great leader you are or aspire to become.

Today in healthcare we are faced with an onslaught of national initiatives. All competing for the same resources, physician leaders have decisions to make about Meaningful Use of Electronic Health Records, clinical integration, accountable care organizations, ICD-10, end of life, quality of care, , and privacy issues among many others. Embodied within all of these efforts is the increasing need for greater consumer and patient engagement. How we measure progress, how we make decisions, and how we take lessons learned from the past to build a bridge to a better place for our hospitals, physician practices and stakeholders in the community ecosystems is the essence of our leadership focus today. Improving the quality of life for all those who live in our communities and seek our organization's help with their comprehensive health and wellness should be a high priority for every physician leader.

By no means is *The Six P's of Physician Leadership* a comprehensive work nor is it intended to be. Instead it is a primer on a complex topic—the nature of being a physician leader in the twenty-first century.

Let this serve as a springboard or a validation metric of your own journey to leadership mastery. We leave you with a final quote. Bill George, in his 2007 work, *True North. Discover Your Authentic Leadership*,

> 'When you are aligned with who you are, you find coherence between your life story and your leadership."[xiv]

As leaders in healthcare today and for the future of the American healthcare system, remember to understand yourself and how you can capitalize on your strengths for the benefit of those around you. Recognize your weaknesses and continuously seek ways to improve your own traits, skills and abilities. The journey is never over, as much like Maslow's hierarchy, ascending to the highest levels is indeed a lifelong and career long quest.

CLOSING THOUGHTS FOR EMERGING LEADERS

In the development of this book a focus was placed on the emerging physician leader and providing a structure for how to grow and develop in ways that matter. There are three additional areas to introduce as advanced considerations for existing leaders that go beyond a simple primer on leadership development.

1. **Governance**—operating at the board level,
2. **Career management**—burnout and long-range career considerations,
3. **Personal work life balance**—not an accidental occurrence.

Relevant application of the *Six P's of Physician Leadership* can be found throughout each of these three advanced considerations. As your own journey unfolds consider each of them.

Governance

Governance—operating at the board level

Many physician leaders emerge because of their innate abilities to lead or because of their credibility as trusted clinicians and colleagues. Some of you have sat on various boards and participated at various levels of engagement.

Taking this up a notch, what about staffing the board? What about setting the agenda and selecting the chairperson, coaching them to success, staffing the meeting and tending to the between meeting relationship needs of board members and stakeholders?

The fundamentals of this book provide the essentials you need to operate in this space. However, recognize that physician leaders are not always taken seriously at the board level in the business of medicine. You must earn your stripes and demonstrate your ability to drive to execution whatever you commit to in terms of goals, objectives and strategic relations. Furthermore boards need to remain focused on organizational oversight and not management. Far too often physicians want to immerse themselves in the details of operations and lose sight of their role in strategic governance. Setting boundaries, maintaining strategic alliances, remaining vigilant of national and regional industry trends, and developing a national network of peers and consultative advisors are critical to operating at the board level and contributing to the governance of any organization.

Career Management

Career management—burnout and long-range career considerations

It has been said that one should be careful what they wish for, as they may get it and wish they hadn't. Some physicians move from clinical medicine to full-time administration and miss the 'simplicity' of patient care or the one-to-one human interaction of direct clinical care. Others thrive in this space. Many physician leaders will continue to be practicing clinicians while some will aspire to make the complete transition. As an industry, all varieties of physician leaders are needed.

In all of those scenarios, recognizing the importance of managing your own career is worth additional consideration for every physician. There are many factors to consider in career management and far too many variations to easily summarize in a few short paragraphs. Each individual scenario is unique and professional coaches should be engaged regardless of your career level. Like any good business plan, if you begin with what you are trying to accomplish and work backwards, you can start to put a timeline down with achievable goals and objectives.

Educational gaps, income and retirement, career shift considerations, geographic limitations, and family dynamics all play into managing one's career. There is no single recipe for getting it right other than to intentionally plan for the future and the most meaningful path rather than leave it to chance.

Burnout is a second component of career management. Perhaps being too successful in your day job, or just ignoring the rest of your life. It has been said that the opposite of happiness is boredom as noted by Timothy Ferriss in his 2009 book, *The 4-Hour Workweek: Escape 9-5, Live Anywhere, and Join the New Rich*.[xv] Don't become so successful that you become bored or worse yet deflated, burned out or even fulminantly depressed. Continually reinventing yourself and staying invigorated are not accidental activities. So let's discuss one approach to having and managing a balanced life.

Work-Life Balance

Personal work life balance – no accidental activity

Achieving business success as a leader is based upon your foundational ability to achieve personal excellence in your life. While many leaders have existed with imbalances and certainly more will come, it seems prudent to at least try to attain success in both.

Without achievable and realistic goals it can be difficult to navigate your way through the forest of life and achieve success at work and your personal life.

For years in my past physician training programs we have taught the elements of a balanced life to residents to help them achieve personal excellence in all that they do. We believe there are no less than six elements of *well-being* and a successful life as listed below.

1. Physical—Health and physical condition

2. Social—Home and family

3. Professional—Life's work or career

4. Financial—Retirement or income goals

5. Emotional-Mental and personal growth

6. Spiritual—Self-fulfillment or spirituality

Each of the six elements of well-being, when attended to with great intention, increases your likelihood of experiencing a fulfilling life. In John B. Izzo's 2004 work, *Second Innocence. Rediscovering Joy and Wonder*, Dr. Izzo talks about "wake up calls" and asks the question "how do we become clear on what is truly important to us?"[xvi] As a physician growing in your career at any stage, remember not to lose sight of this question and within the answer lies some combination of a focus on these six elements of a balanced life.

Physical well-being means tending to your personal wellness. Don't neglect your teeth, get your immunizations, practice a healthy lifestyle through healthy eating, exercise and avoid smoking, for example. All things physicians should be well versed in and should be teaching their patients.

Social well-being includes your home and family life. Do you spend time with your spouse, your children, your extended family?

Do you have one or more close personal friendships? The old adage, "I never met a man, who upon his death bed, wished he had spent more time at work." The survival rule of threes tells us you can survive 3 minutes without air, 3 hours without shelter, 3 days without water, 3 weeks without food, and 3 months without social interaction. Yes, social well-being is essential to your very survival let alone happiness.

Professional well-being is what much of this book has been focused on for emerging and developing leaders. You must tend to your basic competencies, ongoing education and training to maintain your professional well-being.

Financial well-being includes having a financial plan. Retirement planning, college tuition, insurance, long and short-term investments, income targets and charitable contributions are but a glimpse of what this entails.

Emotional well-being includes your personal development beyond your job or profession. What do you do to grow and develop yourself emotionally? Do you have hobbies? Do you travel, study other cultures, read, write, teach, or engage in other activities that keep you sharp and engaged?

Finally, what about your *spiritual well-being*? For some people this entails going to church on Sundays. For others it is about service to others or about meditation or prayer. For some people this is hiking in the woods and communing with nature. Whether mission based or soul searching, it is something to be tended to in your own way and not to be neglected.

Part of becoming a great leader is about personal life management and keeping your own affairs in order. An internal drive to ascend in leadership stirs within each and every person reading this book (or else you would not have read this far). The principles discussed here can apply to leadership across multiple industries and perhaps this closing discussion around life management surprises you but it is an easily overlooked issue and a critical element at the core of being what you wish to become.

Stay vigilant in your own personal journey and please send us your thoughts, testimonials or your suggestions for our next writing on critical needs for today's physician leaders and those in the next generation.

Making the principles and concepts in this book more available and meaningful for our future leaders is a high priority and important for helping meet the challenges that come with the systemic changes occurring in the U.S. and global healthcare system in the twenty-first century.

Visit us at www.6psleadership.com. Your comments and thoughts are welcomed.

BIBLIOGRAPHY

Chabris, C. and Simons, D. *The Invisible Gorilla: How Our Intuitions Deceive Us.* New York, NY: Crown Publishers. 2010.

Christensen C, Grossman JH, Hwang J. *The Innovator's Prescription. A Disruptive Solution for Health Care.* New York, NY: McGraw Hill. 2009.

Collins, J. *Good to Great: why some companies make the leap…and others don't.* New York, NY: HarperCollins Publishers, Inc. 2001.

Covey, SMR. *The Speed of Trust: The One Thing That Changes Everything.* New York, NY: Free Press. 2008.

Crosson FJ, Leu J, Roemer BM, Ross MN. Gaps in residency training should be addressed to better prepare doctors for a twenty-first-century delivery system. *Health Aff (Millwood).* 2011 Nov:30(11);2142-8.

Duberman T, Bloom L. Conard S, and Fromer L. A call for physician leadership at all levels. *Physician Exec.* 2013 Mar-Apr;39(2):24-

6, 28, 30.

Ferriss T. *The 4-Hour Workweek: Escape 9-5, Live Anywhere, and Join the new Rich.* New York, NY: Harmony Books. 2009.

Flareau B, Yale K, Bohn JM, Conschak C. *Clinical Integration. A Roadmap to Accountable Care.* Second Edition. Virginia Beach, VA: Convurgent Publishing. 2011.

George B. *True North. Discover Your Authentic Leadership.* Hoboken, NJ: John Wiley & Sons, Inc. 2007.

Gladwell M. *The Tipping Point. How Little Things Can Make a Big Difference.* New York, NY: Back Bay Books. 2001.

Izzo JB. *Second Innocence. Rediscovering Joy and Wonder.* San Francisco, CA: Berrett-Koehler Publishers, Inc. 2004.

Jaworksi, J. *Synchronicity. The Inner Path of Leadership.* San Francisco, CA: Berrett-Koehler Publishers. 1996.

Patterson, K, Grenny, J, McMillan R, Switzler A. *Crucial Conversations: Tools for Talking When stakes are High.* Second Edition. Columbus,

OH: McGraw-Hill. 2011.

Porter ME and Teisberg EO. *Redefining Health Care. Creating Value-Based Competition on Results.* Boston, MA: Harvard Business School Press. 2006.

Starr P. *The Transformation of American Medicine.* New York, NY: HarperCollins Publishers. 1982.

INDEX

A

accountable care organizations, 62, 75
achievable goals, 83
ACO, 63
    regulatory burdens, 63
American College of Physician Executives, 67

B

Baby Boomers, 22
business acumen, 49

C

Career management, 79, 81
    burnout, 82
Chabris, Christopher, 53
characteristics of paradigm shifts, 62
Christensen, Clayton, 69
clinical integration, 75
collaboration driven, 49
Collins, Jim, 9, 16
communication tool
    instant messaging, 37
    social media, 37
communications, 67
community ecosystem, 76
complex adaptive system, 21

ethical character, 30

F

Facebook, 38
Ferriss, Timothy, 83
Flareau, Donald G., 32
   character, 32
formative feedback, 13

G

George, Bill, 18, 76
Gladwell, Malcolm, 62
Goethe, 10
Good to Great, 9
Governance, 79
   setting boundaries, 81

H

Hackett, Paul, 60
health care reform, 3, 64
Himalayan Rescue Association, 60
Hulu, 38
human behavior, 61
human interaction, 10
humility, 19

I

ICD-10, 75
influence management, 8

MBA, 66
Meaningful Use, 75
medical schools, 2
moral convictions, 33
Mount Everest, 60
multidisciplinary team, 7
Myers Briggs personality inventory, 31

N

names, 15
negotiation, 7

O

one-to-one relationships, 12
operating room, xii
organizational transformation, 1

P

Paine, Thomas, 25
parallel tracking, 54
Patch Adams, 58
patient engagement, 75
patient satisfaction, 70
Patterson, Kerry, 14
perceived character, 38
personal disclosures, 19
perspective, 58
physician leader
    adaptability, 61

[i] Crosson FJ, Leu J, Roemer BM, Ross MN. Gaps in residency training should be addressed to better prepare doctors for a twenty-first-century delivery system. *Health Aff (Millwood)*. 2011 Nov:30(11);2142-8.

[ii] Duberman T, Bloom L. Conard S, and Fromer L. A call for physician leadership at all levels. *Physician Exec.* 2013 Mar-Apr;39(2):24-6, 28, 30

[iii] Collins, J. *Good to Great: why some companies make the leap…and others don't.* New York, NY: HarperCollins Publishers, Inc. 2001.

[iv] Covey, SMR. *The Speed of Trust: The One Thing That Changes Everything.* New York, NY: Free Press. 2008.

ENDNOTES

[v] Patterson, K, Grenny, J, McMillan R, Switzler A. *Crucial Conversations: Tools for Talking When stakes are High.* Second Edition. Columbus, OH: McGraw-Hill. 2011.

[vi] George, B. Knowing Your Authentic Self. In: *True North. Discover Your Authentic Leadership.* San Francisco, CA: Jossey-Bass. 2007. 76.

[vii] Flareau B, Yale K, Bohn JM, Conschak C. The Lens of Leadership. In: *Clinical Integration. A Roadmap to Accountable Care.* Second Edition. Virginia Beach, VA: Convurgent Publishing. 2011. 64-66.

[viii] Chabris, C. and Simons, D. *The Invisible Gorilla: How Our Intuitions Deceive Us.* New York, NY: Crown Publishers. 2010.

[ix] Gladwell M. Introduction. In: *The Tipping*

Point. How Little Things Can Make a Big Difference. New York, NY: Back Bay Books. 2001. 9.

[x] Jaworksi, J. Creating the Future. In: *Synchronicity. The Inner Path of Leadership.* San Francisco, CA: Berrett-Koehler Publishers. 1996. 185.

[xi] Christensen C, Grossman JH, Hwang J. Introduction. In: *The Innovator's Prescription. A Disruptive Solution for Health Care.* New York, NY: McGraw Hill. 2009. xx.

[xii] Porter ME and Teisberg EO. Introduction. In: *Redefining Health Care. Creating Value-Based Competition on Results.* Boston, MA: Harvard Business School Press. 2006. 15.

[xiii] Starr P. The Social Origins of Professional Sovereignty. In: *The Transformation of American Medicine.* New York, NY: HarperCollins Publishers. 1982. 5.

[xiv] George B. Introduction. In: *True North. Discover Your Authentic Leadership.* Hoboken, NJ: John Wiley & Sons, Inc. 2007. xxiv.

[xv] Ferriss T. *The 4-Hour Workweek: Escape 9-5, Live Anywhere, and Join the new Rich.* New York, NY: Harmony Books. 2009.

[xvi] Izzo JB. Full speed Ahead in the Wrong Direction. In: *Second Innocence. Rediscovering Joy and Wonder.* San Francisco, CA: Berrett-Koehler Publishers, Inc., 2004. 27.

Page intentionally left blank

39363695R00065

Made in the USA
Lexington, KY
20 February 2015